4 seasons in 4 weeks

4s4w Daily Tracker and Journal

Suzanne Mathis McQueen

Tobacco Road Press
Ashland, Oregon

Copyright©2012 by Suzanne Mathis McQueen

ISBN: 978-0-9858955-1-8

Four Seasons in Four Weeks® is a registered trademark

Published by Tobacco Road Press

Ashland, Oregon

Printed in China

Editor: Jessica Vineyard, Red Letter Editing

Interior Design: Christy Collins, Confluence Book Services

Book Cover: Gaelyn Larrick

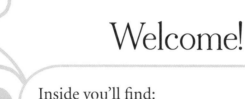

Welcome!

Inside you'll find:

1) Instructions for Weekly Tracker Tables

2) Weekly Tracker Tables

3) Instructions for Daily Trackers

4) Two months of Daily Tracker pages, specific to each seasonal week

5) Daily Journal

6) Instructions for Monthly Tracker Table

7) Monthly Tracker Table

8) Instructions for reordering

This Tracker and Journal is designed to be used in conjunction with my book, *4 Seasons in 4 Weeks*. Tracking your cycle is the best way to get in tune with your monthly rhythm. My suggestion is to refer to the book for detailed descriptions, reminders, to-dos, and more, especially once you start seeing the patterns in your unique rhythm. Track for at least three months to tune in to what is natural for you. There are three different options for tracking: daily, weekly, and monthly. I encourage you to use the easiest and most enjoyable method for you. You may find that, like me, you want to continue tracking your cycle indefinitely in order to stay focused on your personal well-being, that of your family, and the world community.

–In good nature, Suzanne

Instructions for Tracking Your Cycle

Tracking your cycle is easy and meant to be an enjoyable experience. Tuning in to your monthly rhythm is an opportunity to reveal your Authentic Female and provides a designated time each day to do something luxurious for yourself.

There are three Tracking Charts in this Daily Tracker and Journal: Daily, Weekly, and Monthly. Use one, two, or all three. I suggest you begin with the Daily Tracker in order to get the hang of tracking. Download the free, full-size Monthly Tracker at 4seasons4weeks.com.

Tracking by hormones: This is for cycling women. Day 1 is the first full day of your Period.

Tracking by the Moon: This is for women who are no longer bleeding. Day 1 starts on the New Moon. Follow along with the phases of the Moon; each chart will therefore be used for only seven days. Leave the last two days blank and move on to the next Weekly Tracker.

Using the Weekly Tracker

The Weekly Tracker is a quick reference guide and overview of your monthly cycle. It can be used alone or in conjunction with the Daily Tracker.

Before you go to bed at night, reflect upon your day and take a couple of minutes to mark the boxes on the chart. On the upper section of categories, use a minus (—), zero (O), or plus (+) to indicate low/poor, medium/neutral, or high/great to describe how you're feeling in the category indicated. For instance, if your overall health feels great, then mark "+" in the appropriate box for that day. In the lower section, use an "X" to mark a box when that particular indicator rings true for you that day. Feel free to make your own identifying marks—whatever makes it easier for you to read your own chart.

Categories:

Month: Enter the current month(s) you are tracking; for instance, June/July.

Date: Enter the calendar day. For instance, you might begin your Period on June 7th, so your Date boxes would look like 7, 8, 9, etc.

4s4w Cycle Day #: This shows how the days are figured in the standard 4s4w strategy of seven days per seasonal week. Your cycle may look just like it, or not. You won't be marking in these boxes.

My Cycle Day #: This is where you track your unique cycle. Begin Week 1, Fall with (Day) 1 as the first day of your Period, then, 2, 3, etc. If, for instance, your Fall week lasts for six days, then begin Week 2, Winter with (Day) 7, 8, 9.

Use the symbols —, O, + for low/poor, medium/neutral, or high/great

Here is what you'll rate:

> **Overall Health:** How you're generally feeling
>
> **Energy:** High or low
>
> **Libido:** Sex drive
>
> **Mind Mood:** Mental/emotional outlook or viewpoint
>
> **Sleep:** Good or restless
>
> **Communication:** How well you are communicating with others
>
> **Self-esteem:** How you are feeling about yourself

On the following, mark an "X" if it applies, leave blank if not

> **Contraception:** Did you use it?
>
> **Sex:** Did you have it?

Exercise: Did you get some in?

Good nutrition: Did you eat well?

Beauty/Self-care: Did you get your hair cut or take a long bubble bath? Use a scale of 1–10

Feeling the Love: How much love are you feeling toward others or yourself? Use a scale of 1–10

INDICATORS: Use an "X" to indicate whether you experienced this on a particular day. Fill in blanks at the bottom of the chart with your own indicators, if desired.

Daily Tracker and Journal

Upon waking, take a moment to notice the week and the cycle day you are on and what they mean with respect to your self-care. Do you need to be resting, building relationships, fully expressing, or fire walking? Please refer to the *4 Seasons in 4 Weeks* book for more information about the week you are on.

1) Fill out the "morning" section of the Tracker. Choose an intention for the day. For example, you may enter "eating well." A "strength" word indicates a particular super-trait you'd like to have support you, such as courage or grace. "Why" helps you focus on your desired outcome. "My intention is to focus on eating well (why) because my body feels better when I do." "My strength word today is 'ability' (why) because I'm learning to manage my finances well." *See word suggestions on page 7.*

2) Fill in the "evening" section before retiring at night. Write one or more words in each box to describe what you're feeling. For example, under "Power" you might write "awesome!"

3) Use the lined page at any time to journal about your day.

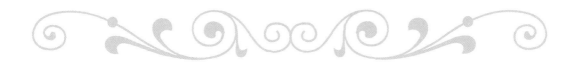

Examples of Intention for the Day

Eat well. Play with partner/kids. Exercise 30 minutes. Smile at everyone. Meet two new people. Pamper myself. Rest. Let go of guilt. Write a letter. Read a book. Be calm. Forgive someone. Stay present.

Examples of Strength Words

Courage, fearlessness, grace, truth, wisdom, power, beauty, ability, adventure, artistry, motivation, generosity, compassion, success, comfort, confidence, forgiveness, focus, perfection.

Examples of Descriptive Words for Daily Tracker Boxes

Choose one or two words for each box. Feel free to make your own list! Find your voice!

Solid, centered, inconsistent, fragile, unfocused, in tune, accessed, stumbled, passed down, appreciated, confident, growing, not present, tenuous, glowing, radiant, luminous, affectionate, sensuous, sexual, expansive, irritable, loud, soft, quiet, internal, external, cozy, depressed, happy, not happy, vulnerable, mad, gorgeous, enlightened, stuck, dismissed, lightened load, playful, energetic, sluggish, I WANT CHOCOLATE!

Adjusting the amount of days in a week for your unique rhythm: Weekly and Daily Trackers

Every woman's cycle is unique to her. The 4s4w system breaks down the approximately 28 days into four guided weeks of seven days each. This is simply a beginning template. You may discover that your Week 1, Fall is five days long and your Week 2, Winter is nine days long, or vice versa. The Trackers have nine days in each week if you need them. The mysteries of your body, mind, and soul will come into focus when you tap in to your experience and keep track of it over a period of time.

Defining, adjusting, and transitioning from one seasonal week to the next:

Please review each seasonal week in the book, *4 Seasons in 4 Weeks*, prior to starting each of your cycle weeks.

Week 1, Fall begins on the first day of your Period. Mark each day that you bleed. Once you are done bleeding, evaluate whether you still need rest or if you're feeling energetic and anxious to move into the next seasonal week. Week 1 will vary greatly among women. You may have a five-day week or an eight-day week. Once you feel complete, abandon the rest of the days on the chart and move on to the next one, Week 2, Winter. The more months you track, the better you'll get at assessing your rhythm.

Week 2, Winter begins the first day your mind shifts from planning to doing and your physical body feels ready to shift from internal to external. It's a little like sitting in a car for too long on a road trip and needing to stretch your legs.

Week 3, Spring begins with Ovulation. Please see the Ovulation section in the book. You'll either be making a guesstimation, using an Ovulation kit, or counting birth control pills. If you are on the Pill you won't ovulate, but your hormones will still rise and your body will still want to fully express itself.

Week 4, Summer begins when your body goes from feeling calm and energetic to electrically charged, on edge, with rumbling energy inside. You might feel the need to "burn off energy."

Enjoy tracking your rhythm. Get into it! You may find that you develop a lifelong habit as you tune in to YOU.

Month									
Begin this week at Cyclers: The Period Non-Cyclers: New Moon	Week 1, Fall Period New Moon Rest ❧ Receive ❧ Rejuvenate Internal								
Date									
4s4w Cycle Day #	1	2	3	4	5	6	7		
My Cycle Day #									
Low — Med O High +									
Overall Health — O +									
Energy — O +									
Libido — O +									
Mind Mood — O +									
Sleep — O +									
Communication — O +									
Self-Esteem — O +									
Contraception									
Sex									
Exercise									
Good nutrition									
Beauty/Self-care 1–10									
Feeling the Love 1–10									
Indicators									
Headache									
Acne									
Cramps 1–10									
Breast tenderness									
Irritability									
Depression									
Appetite/Cravings									
Rest									
Visions/Ideas									
Artwork									

Month									
Begin this week at Cyclers: Period over and feeling active Non-Cyclers: 1st Quarter Moon	Week 2, Winter Venus Week Waxing Gibbous Moon Become ✍ Connect ✍ Attract External								
Date									
4s4w Cycle Day #	8	9	10	11	12	13	14		
My Cycle Day #									
Low — Med O High +									
Overall Health — O +									
Energy — O +									
Libido — O +									
Mind Mood — O +									
Sleep — O +									
Communication — O +									
Self-Esteem — O +									
Contraception									
Sex									
Exercise									
Good nutrition									
Beauty/Self-care 1–10									
Feeling the Love 1–10									
Indicators									
Headache									
Irritability									
Depression									
Connect with friends									
Connect with partner									
Project building									
Play									

Month										
Begin this week at Cyclers: Ovulation Non-Cyclers: Full Moon	Week 3, Spring Ovulation Full Moon Fully Express ⤎ Lead External									
Date										
4s4w Cycle Day #	15	16	17	18	19	20	21			
My Cycle Day #										
Low — Med O High +										
Overall Health — O +										
Energy — O +										
Libido — O +										
Mind Mood — O +										
Sleep — O +										
Communication — O +										
Self-Esteem — O +										
Contraception										
Sex										
Exercise										
Good Nutrition										
Beauty/Self-care 1–10										
Feeling the Love 1–10										
Indicators										
Headache										
Irritability										
Identified Ovulation										
Depression										
Reflect/Evaluate Life										
Leadership 1–10										
Full Expression + — O										

Month										
Begin this week at Cyclers: Smooth high energy becomes edgy Non-Cyclers: 3rd Quarter Moon	Week 4, Summer Fire Walk Waning Crescent Moon Burn off energy ↝ Observe ↝ Overcome Internal									
Date										
4s4w Cycle Day #	22	23	24	25	26	27	28			
My Cycle Day #										
Low — Med O High +										
Overall Health — O +										
Energy — O +										
Libido — O +										
Mind Mood — O +										
Sleep — O +										
Communication — O +										
Self-Esteem — O +										
Contraception										
Sex										
Exercise										
Good nutrition										
Beauty/Self-care 1–10										
Feeling the Love 1–10										
Indicators										
Headache										
Acne										
Cramps 1–10										
Breast tenderness										
Irritability										
Depression										
"Hot Spots"										
Intensity 1–10										
Organizing										
Meditation										

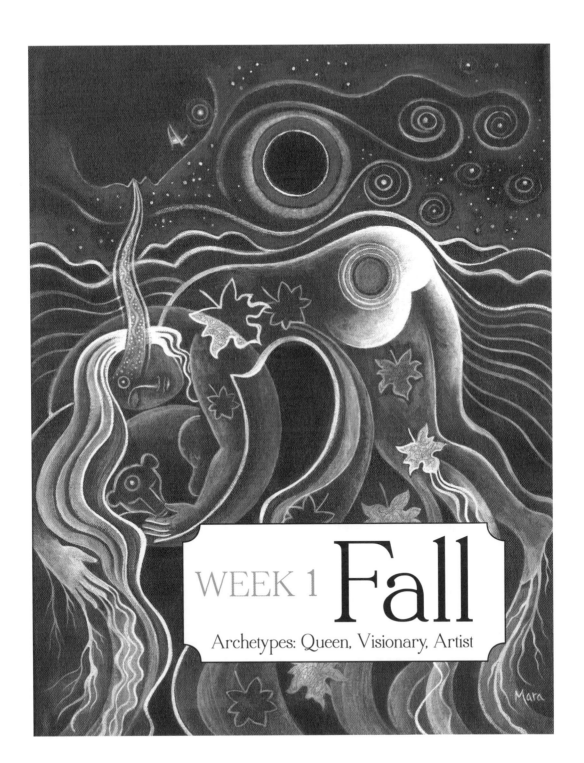

WEEK 1 Fall

Archetypes: Queen, Visionary, Artist

Daily Tracker — Week 1, Fall

Cycle Day: _____ Date: _____ Focus: Rest ☙ Receive ☙ Rejuvenate

MORNING

Woke up feeling: _____

Intention for the day: _____

Strength for the day: _____

Why? _____

EVENING

Physical Energy	Libido	Mind Mood
Blood Flow	I'm letting go of…	Challenges
Rest	Visions/Ideas/Seedlings	Artwork/Creativity/Ritual
Power	Wisdom	Inner Beauty

JOURNAL

Daily Tracker — Week 1, Fall

Cycle Day: _____ Date: _____ Focus: Rest ⚜ Receive ⚜ Rejuvenate

MORNING

Woke up feeling: _____

Intention for the day: _____

Strength for the day: _____

Why? _____

EVENING

Physical Energy	Libido	Mind Mood
Blood Flow	I'm letting go of…	Challenges
Rest	Visions/Ideas/Seedlings	Artwork/Creativity/Ritual
Power	Wisdom	Inner Beauty

JOURNAL

Daily Tracker — Week 1, Fall

Cycle Day: _____ Date: _____ Focus: Rest ❧ Receive ❧ Rejuvenate

MORNING

Woke up feeling: _____

Intention for the day: _____

Strength for the day: _____

Why? _____

EVENING

Physical Energy	Libido	Mind Mood
Blood Flow	I'm letting go of…	Challenges
Rest	Visions/Ideas/Seedlings	Artwork/Creativity/Ritual
Power	Wisdom	Inner Beauty

JOURNAL

Daily Tracker — Week 1, Fall

Cycle Day: _____ Date: _____ Focus: Rest ☙ Receive ☙ Rejuvenate

MORNING

Woke up feeling: _____

Intention for the day: _____

Strength for the day: _____

Why? _____

EVENING

Physical Energy	Libido	Mind Mood
Blood Flow	I'm letting go of…	Challenges
Rest	Visions/Ideas/Seedlings	Artwork/Creativity/Ritual
Power	Wisdom	Inner Beauty

JOURNAL

Daily Tracker — Week 1, Fall

Cycle Day: _____ Date: _____ Focus: Rest ⚜ Receive ⚜ Rejuvenate

MORNING

Woke up feeling: _____

Intention for the day: _____

Strength for the day: _____

Why? _____

EVENING

Physical Energy	Libido	Mind Mood
Blood Flow	I'm letting go of...	Challenges
Rest	Visions/Ideas/Seedlings	Artwork/Creativity/Ritual
Power	Wisdom	Inner Beauty

JOURNAL

Daily Tracker — Week 1, Fall

Cycle Day: _____ Date: _____ Focus: Rest ✿ Receive ✿ Rejuvenate

MORNING

Woke up feeling: _____

Intention for the day: _____

Strength for the day: _____

Why? _____

EVENING

Physical Energy	Libido	Mind Mood
Blood Flow	I'm letting go of…	Challenges
Rest	Visions/Ideas/Seedlings	Artwork/Creativity/Ritual
Power	Wisdom	Inner Beauty

JOURNAL

Daily Tracker — Week 1, Fall

Cycle Day: _____ Date: _____ Focus: Rest ❧ Receive ❧ Rejuvenate

MORNING

Woke up feeling: _____

Intention for the day: _____

Strength for the day: _____

Why? _____

EVENING

Physical Energy	Libido	Mind Mood
Blood Flow	I'm letting go of…	Challenges
Rest	Visions/Ideas/Seedlings	Artwork/Creativity/Ritual
Power	Wisdom	Inner Beauty

JOURNAL

Daily Tracker — Week 1, Fall

Cycle Day: _____ Date: _____ Focus: Rest ❧ Receive ❧ Rejuvenate

MORNING

Woke up feeling: _____

Intention for the day: _____

Strength for the day: _____

Why? _____

EVENING

Physical Energy	Libido	Mind Mood
Blood Flow	I'm letting go of…	Challenges
Rest	Visions/Ideas/Seedlings	Artwork/Creativity/Ritual
Power	Wisdom	Inner Beauty

JOURNAL

Daily Tracker — Week 1, Fall

Cycle Day: _____ Date: _____ Focus: Rest ❦ Receive ❦ Rejuvenate

MORNING

Woke up feeling: _____

Intention for the day: _____

Strength for the day: _____

Why? _____

EVENING

Physical Energy	Libido	Mind Mood
Blood Flow	I'm letting go of...	Challenges
Rest	Visions/Ideas/Seedlings	Artwork/Creativity/Ritual
Power	Wisdom	Inner Beauty

JOURNAL

NOTES

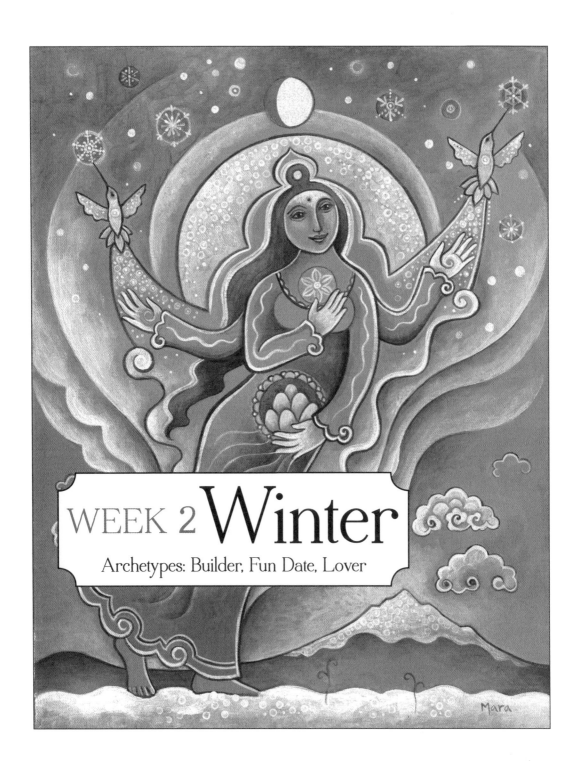

WEEK 2 Winter

Archetypes: Builder, Fun Date, Lover

Daily Tracker — Week 2, Winter

Cycle Day:____ Date:_____ Focus: Become ⚜ Connect ⚜ Attract

MORNING

Woke up feeling: _____

Intention for the day: _____

Strength for the day: _____

Why? _____

EVENING

Physical Energy	Libido	Mind Mood
Heart-to-Heart Talks	Beauty Regimen	Challenges
Connections: People or Projects	Fun Outings	Obsessions
Power	Wisdom	Inner Beauty

JOURNAL

Daily Tracker — Week 2, Winter

Cycle Day:_____ Date:_____ Focus: Become ❧ Connect ❧ Attract

MORNING

Woke up feeling: _____

Intention for the day: _____

Strength for the day: _____

Why? _____

EVENING

Physical Energy	Libido	Mind Mood
Heart-to-Heart Talks	Beauty Regimen	Challenges
Connections: People or Projects	Fun Outings	Obsessions
Power	Wisdom	Inner Beauty

JOURNAL

Daily Tracker — Week 2, Winter

Cycle Day:____ Date:_____ Focus: Become ☙ Connect ☙ Attract

MORNING

Woke up feeling: _____

Intention for the day: _____

Strength for the day: _____

Why? _____

EVENING

Physical Energy	Libido	Mind Mood
Heart-to-Heart Talks	Beauty Regimen	Challenges
Connections: People or Projects	Fun Outings	Obsessions
Power	Wisdom	Inner Beauty

JOURNAL

Daily Tracker — Week 2, Winter

Cycle Day: _____ Date: _____ Focus: Become ❧ Connect ❧ Attract

MORNING

Woke up feeling: _____

Intention for the day: _____

Strength for the day: _____

Why? _____

EVENING

Physical Energy	Libido	Mind Mood
Heart-to-Heart Talks	Beauty Regimen	Challenges
Connections: People or Projects	Fun Outings	Obsessions
Power	Wisdom	Inner Beauty

JOURNAL

Daily Tracker — Week 2, Winter

Cycle Day:____ Date:_____   Focus: Become ॐ Connect ॐ Attract

MORNING

Woke up feeling: _____

Intention for the day: _____

Strength for the day: _____

Why? _____

EVENING

Physical Energy	Libido	Mind Mood
Heart-to-Heart Talks	Beauty Regimen	Challenges
Connections: People or Projects	Fun Outings	Obsessions
Power	Wisdom	Inner Beauty

JOURNAL

Daily Tracker — Week 2, Winter

Cycle Day: ____ Date: _____ Focus: Become ❧ Connect ❧ Attract

MORNING

Woke up feeling: _____

Intention for the day: _____

Strength for the day: _____

Why? _____

EVENING

Physical Energy	Libido	Mind Mood
Heart-to-Heart Talks	Beauty Regimen	Challenges
Connections: People or Projects	Fun Outings	Obsessions
Power	Wisdom	Inner Beauty

JOURNAL

Daily Tracker — Week 2, Winter

Cycle Day:____ Date:_____ Focus: Become ❧ Connect ❧ Attract

MORNING

Woke up feeling: _____

Intention for the day: _____

Strength for the day: _____

Why? _____

EVENING

Physical Energy	Libido	Mind Mood
Heart-to-Heart Talks	Beauty Regimen	Challenges
Connections: People or Projects	Fun Outings	Obsessions
Power	Wisdom	Inner Beauty

JOURNAL

Daily Tracker — Week 2, Winter

Cycle Day:____ Date:_____ Focus: Become ❧ Connect ❧ Attract

MORNING

Woke up feeling: _____

Intention for the day: _____

Strength for the day: _____

Why? _____

EVENING

Physical Energy	Libido	Mind Mood
Heart-to-Heart Talks	Beauty Regimen	Challenges
Connections: People or Projects	Fun Outings	Obsessions
Power	Wisdom	Inner Beauty

JOURNAL

Daily Tracker — Week 2, Winter

Cycle Day: ____ Date: _____ Focus: Become ✤ Connect ✤ Attract

MORNING

Woke up feeling: _____

Intention for the day: _____

Strength for the day: _____

Why? _____

EVENING

Physical Energy	Libido	Mind Mood
Heart-to-Heart Talks	Beauty Regimen	Challenges
Connections: People or Projects	Fun Outings	Obsessions
Power	Wisdom	Inner Beauty

JOURNAL

NOTES

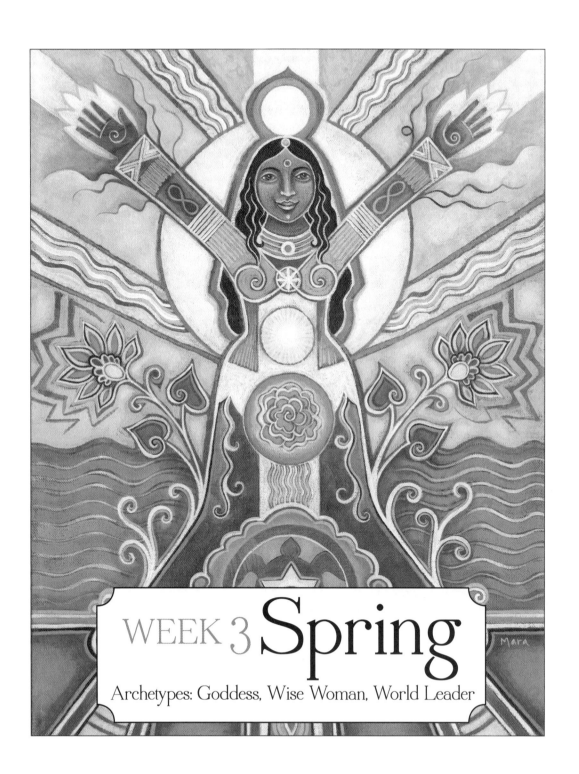

WEEK 3 Spring

Archetypes: Goddess, Wise Woman, World Leader

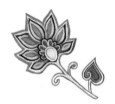

Daily Tracker — Week 3, Spring

Cycle Day: _____ Date: _____ Focus: Fully Express & Lead

MORNING

Woke up feeling: _____

Intention for the day: _____

Strength for the day: _____

Why? _____

EVENING

Physical Energy	Libido	Mind Mood
Full Expression	Vulnerability	Challenges
Authenticity	Mothering	Leadership
Power	Wisdom	Inner Beauty

JOURNAL

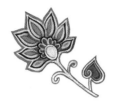

Daily Tracker — Week 3, Spring

Cycle Day: _____ Date: _____ Focus: Fully Express & Lead

MORNING

Woke up feeling: _____

Intention for the day: _____

Strength for the day: _____

Why? _____

EVENING

Physical Energy	Libido	Mind Mood
Full Expression	Vulnerability	Challenges
Authenticity	Mothering	Leadership
Power	Wisdom	Inner Beauty

JOURNAL

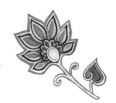

Daily Tracker — Week 3, Spring

Cycle Day: _____ Date: _____ Focus: Fully Express & Lead

MORNING

Woke up feeling: _____

Intention for the day: _____

Strength for the day: _____

Why? _____

EVENING

Physical Energy	Libido	Mind Mood
Full Expression	Vulnerability	Challenges
Authenticity	Mothering	Leadership
Power	Wisdom	Inner Beauty

JOURNAL

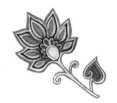

Daily Tracker — Week 3, Spring

Cycle Day: _____ Date: _____ Focus: Fully Express & Lead

MORNING

Woke up feeling: _____

Intention for the day: _____

Strength for the day: _____

Why? _____

EVENING

Physical Energy	Libido	Mind Mood
Full Expression	Vulnerability	Challenges
Authenticity	Mothering	Leadership
Power	Wisdom	Inner Beauty

JOURNAL

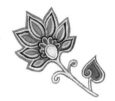

Daily Tracker — Week 3, Spring

Cycle Day: _____ Date: _____ Focus: Fully Express & Lead

MORNING

Woke up feeling: _____

Intention for the day: _____

Strength for the day: _____

Why? _____

EVENING

Physical Energy	Libido	Mind Mood
Full Expression	Vulnerability	Challenges
Authenticity	Mothering	Leadership
Power	Wisdom	Inner Beauty

JOURNAL

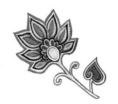

Daily Tracker — Week 3, Spring

Cycle Day: _____ Date: _____ Focus: Fully Express & Lead

MORNING

Woke up feeling: _____

Intention for the day: _____

Strength for the day: _____

Why? _____

EVENING

Physical Energy	Libido	Mind Mood
Full Expression	Vulnerability	Challenges
Authenticity	Mothering	Leadership
Power	Wisdom	Inner Beauty

JOURNAL

Daily Tracker — Week 3, Spring

Cycle Day: _____ Date: _____ Focus: Fully Express & Lead

MORNING

Woke up feeling: _____

Intention for the day: _____

Strength for the day: _____

Why? _____

EVENING

Physical Energy	Libido	Mind Mood
Full Expression	Vulnerability	Challenges
Authenticity	Mothering	Leadership
Power	Wisdom	Inner Beauty

JOURNAL

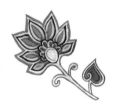

Daily Tracker — Week 3, Spring

Cycle Day: _____ Date: _____ Focus: Fully Express & Lead

MORNING

Woke up feeling: _____

Intention for the day: _____

Strength for the day: _____

Why? _____

EVENING

Physical Energy	Libido	Mind Mood
Full Expression	Vulnerability	Challenges
Authenticity	Mothering	Leadership
Power	Wisdom	Inner Beauty

JOURNAL

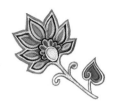

Daily Tracker — Week 3, Spring

Cycle Day: _____ Date: _____ Focus: Fully Express & Lead

MORNING

Woke up feeling: _____

Intention for the day: _____

Strength for the day: _____

Why? _____

EVENING

Physical Energy	Libido	Mind Mood
Full Expression	Vulnerability	Challenges
Authenticity	Mothering	Leadership
Power	Wisdom	Inner Beauty

JOURNAL

NOTES

WEEK 4 Summer
Archetypes: Athlete, Fire Walker, Monk

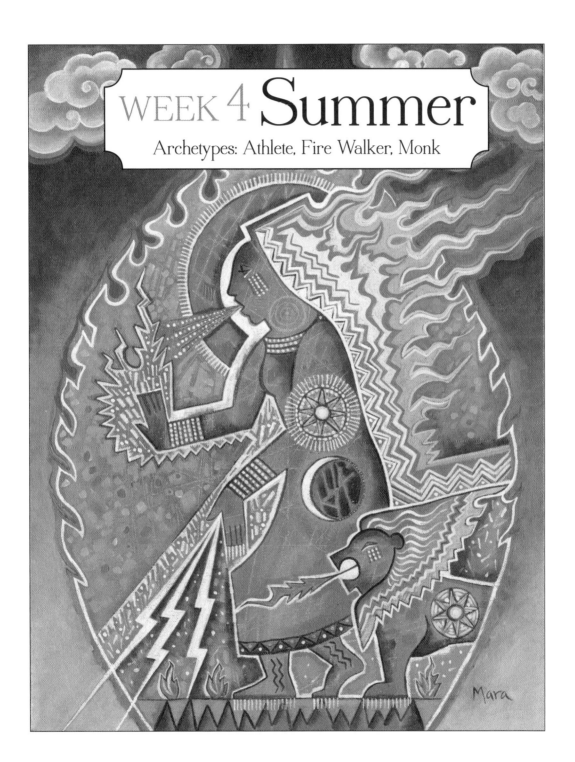

Daily Tracker — Week 4, Summer

Cycle Day:_____ Date:_____ Focus: Exercise ✣ Observe ✣ Overcome

MORNING

Woke up feeling: _____

Intention for the day: _____

Strength for the day: _____

Why? _____

EVENING

Physical Energy	Libido	Mind Mood
Sports	Hot Spots	Challenges
Focus	I'm letting go of…	I'm keeping…
Power	Wisdom	Inner Beauty

JOURNAL

Daily Tracker — Week 4, Summer

Cycle Day:____ Date:_____ Focus: Exercise ❧ Observe ❧ Overcome

MORNING

Woke up feeling: _____

Intention for the day: _____

Strength for the day: _____

Why? _____

EVENING

Physical Energy	Libido	Mind Mood
Sports	Hot Spots	Challenges
Focus	I'm letting go of…	I'm keeping…
Power	Wisdom	Inner Beauty

JOURNAL

Daily Tracker — Week 4, Summer

Cycle Day:____ Date:_____ Focus: Exercise ❀ Observe ❀ Overcome

MORNING

Woke up feeling: _____

Intention for the day: _____

Strength for the day: _____

Why? _____

EVENING

Physical Energy	Libido	Mind Mood
Sports	Hot Spots	Challenges
Focus	I'm letting go of…	I'm keeping…
Power	Wisdom	Inner Beauty

JOURNAL

Daily Tracker — Week 4, Summer

Cycle Day:____ Date:_____ Focus: Exercise ❧ Observe ❧ Overcome

MORNING

Woke up feeling: _____

Intention for the day: _____

Strength for the day: _____

Why? _____

EVENING

Physical Energy	Libido	Mind Mood
Sports	Hot Spots	Challenges
Focus	I'm letting go of...	I'm keeping...
Power	Wisdom	Inner Beauty

JOURNAL

Daily Tracker — Week 4, Summer

Cycle Day:____ Date:_____ Focus: Exercise ॐ Observe ॐ Overcome

MORNING

Woke up feeling: _____

Intention for the day: _____

Strength for the day: _____

Why? _____

EVENING

Physical Energy	Libido	Mind Mood
Sports	Hot Spots	Challenges
Focus	I'm letting go of…	I'm keeping…
Power	Wisdom	Inner Beauty

JOURNAL

Daily Tracker — Week 4, Summer

Cycle Day:____ Date:_____ Focus: Exercise ॐ Observe ॐ Overcome

MORNING

Woke up feeling: _____

Intention for the day: _____

Strength for the day: _____

Why? _____

EVENING

Physical Energy	Libido	Mind Mood
Sports	Hot Spots	Challenges
Focus	I'm letting go of…	I'm keeping…
Power	Wisdom	Inner Beauty

JOURNAL

Daily Tracker — Week 4, Summer

Cycle Day:____ Date:_____ Focus: Exercise ۵ Observe ۵ Overcome

MORNING

Woke up feeling: _____

Intention for the day: _____

Strength for the day: _____

Why? _____

EVENING

Physical Energy	Libido	Mind Mood
Sports	Hot Spots	Challenges
Focus	I'm letting go of…	I'm keeping…
Power	Wisdom	Inner Beauty

JOURNAL

Daily Tracker — Week 4, Summer

Cycle Day:____ Date:_____ Focus: Exercise ❦ Observe ❦ Overcome

MORNING

Woke up feeling: _____

Intention for the day: _____

Strength for the day: _____

Why? _____

EVENING

Physical Energy	Libido	Mind Mood
Sports	Hot Spots	Challenges
Focus	I'm letting go of...	I'm keeping...
Power	Wisdom	Inner Beauty

JOURNAL

Daily Tracker — Week 4, Summer

Cycle Day:____ Date:_____ Focus: Exercise ❧ Observe ❧ Overcome

MORNING

Woke up feeling: _____

Intention for the day: _____

Strength for the day: _____

Why? _____

EVENING

Physical Energy	Libido	Mind Mood
Sports	Hot Spots	Challenges
Focus	I'm letting go of…	I'm keeping…
Power	Wisdom	Inner Beauty

JOURNAL

NOTES

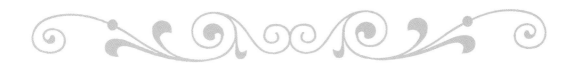

Great! You've just finished your fourth week, Summer. Remember that your cycle is continuous. There's no interruption in your rhythm; feel the flow right into next week, Fall. However, this is a good time to review the last four weeks, consider what you've learned about your rhythm, and prepare for the upcoming four weeks.

Notice how each week has a beginning, a middle, and an end. For instance, **Winter** week begins *after* your Period. Your juices will be drier then, but by the end of **that** week you'll be very wet. With **Spring** week you'll start out very sexual, but after Ovulation your sexuality will take on a new form and continue to morph in beautiful ways.

Start to blend the weeks together by getting in the habit of planning ahead for the following season. For example, if you want to feel better during your **Summer** Fire Walk, then begin making great decisions toward that goal during **Spring** week. A great female recycling experience can be easily attained with mindfulness.

Below are some questions to ask yourself. Also write down any lessons or experiences you had that aren't listed. Remember, this is all about you!

Were your shifts into each seasonal week noticeable? In what ways?

_____
_____
_____
_____

What ideas do you have for preparing for each seasonal week in the upcoming month?

_____
_____
_____
_____

Looking back over the last month, do you see a rhythm in your Mind Moods? If so, how would it help you to watch for this rhythm in the upcoming month?

_____
_____
_____
_____

How will you take care of yourself during your "hot spots?"

_____
_____
_____
_____

It's also time to order your next journal. By doing so now, you won't miss any tracking days. Simply visit www.4seasons4weeks.com to place your order.

Now it's time to cycle into Week 1, Fall. Have a terrific month and enjoy tuning in to your unique feminine rhythm!

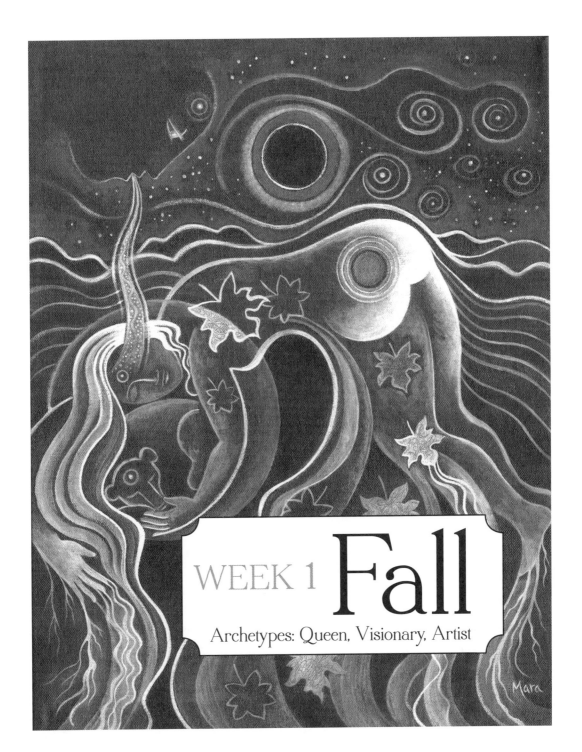

Daily Tracker — Week 1, Fall

Cycle Day: _____ Date: _____ Focus: Rest ☙ Receive ☙ Rejuvenate

MORNING

Woke up feeling: _____

Intention for the day: _____

Strength for the day: _____

Why? _____

EVENING

Physical Energy	Libido	Mind Mood
Blood Flow	I'm letting go of...	Challenges
Rest	Visions/Ideas/Seedlings	Artwork/Creativity/Ritual
Power	Wisdom	Inner Beauty

JOURNAL

Daily Tracker — Week 1, Fall

Cycle Day: _____ Date: _____ Focus: Rest ♦ Receive ♦ Rejuvenate

MORNING

Woke up feeling: _____

Intention for the day: _____

Strength for the day: _____

Why? _____

EVENING

Physical Energy	Libido	Mind Mood
Blood Flow	I'm letting go of…	Challenges
Rest	Visions/Ideas/Seedlings	Artwork/Creativity/Ritual
Power	Wisdom	Inner Beauty

JOURNAL

Daily Tracker — Week 1, Fall

Cycle Day: _____ Date: _____ Focus: Rest ❦ Receive ❦ Rejuvenate

MORNING

Woke up feeling: _____

Intention for the day: _____

Strength for the day: _____

Why? _____

EVENING

Physical Energy	Libido	Mind Mood
Blood Flow	I'm letting go of...	Challenges
Rest	Visions/Ideas/Seedlings	Artwork/Creativity/Ritual
Power	Wisdom	Inner Beauty

JOURNAL

Daily Tracker — Week 1, Fall

Cycle Day: _____ Date: _____ Focus: Rest ⚜ Receive ⚜ Rejuvenate

MORNING

Woke up feeling: _____

Intention for the day: _____

Strength for the day: _____

Why? _____

EVENING

Physical Energy	Libido	Mind Mood
Blood Flow	I'm letting go of…	Challenges
Rest	Visions/Ideas/Seedlings	Artwork/Creativity/Ritual
Power	Wisdom	Inner Beauty

JOURNAL

Daily Tracker — Week 1, Fall

Cycle Day: _____   Date: _____   Focus: Rest ☙ Receive ☙ Rejuvenate

MORNING

Woke up feeling: _____

Intention for the day: _____

Strength for the day: _____

Why? _____

EVENING

Physical Energy	Libido	Mind Mood
Blood Flow	I'm letting go of...	Challenges
Rest	Visions/Ideas/Seedlings	Artwork/Creativity/Ritual
Power	Wisdom	Inner Beauty

JOURNAL

Daily Tracker — Week 1, Fall

Cycle Day: _____   Date: _____   Focus: Rest ࿎ Receive ࿎ Rejuvenate

MORNING

Woke up feeling: _____

Intention for the day: _____

Strength for the day: _____

Why? _____

EVENING

Physical Energy	Libido	Mind Mood
Blood Flow	I'm letting go of…	Challenges
Rest	Visions/Ideas/Seedlings	Artwork/Creativity/Ritual
Power	Wisdom	Inner Beauty

JOURNAL

Daily Tracker — Week 1, Fall

Cycle Day: _____ Date: _____ Focus: Rest ⚘ Receive ⚘ Rejuvenate

MORNING

Woke up feeling: _____

Intention for the day: _____

Strength for the day: _____

Why? _____

EVENING

Physical Energy	Libido	Mind Mood
Blood Flow	I'm letting go of…	Challenges
Rest	Visions/Ideas/Seedlings	Artwork/Creativity/Ritual
Power	Wisdom	Inner Beauty

JOURNAL

Daily Tracker — Week 1, Fall

Cycle Day: _____ Date: _____ Focus: Rest ❧ Receive ❧ Rejuvenate

MORNING

Woke up feeling: _____

Intention for the day: _____

Strength for the day: _____

Why? _____

EVENING

Physical Energy	Libido	Mind Mood
Blood Flow	I'm letting go of…	Challenges
Rest	Visions/Ideas/Seedlings	Artwork/Creativity/Ritual
Power	Wisdom	Inner Beauty

JOURNAL

Daily Tracker — Week 1, Fall

Cycle Day: _____ Date: _____ Focus: Rest ❦ Receive ❦ Rejuvenate

MORNING

Woke up feeling: _____

Intention for the day: _____

Strength for the day: _____

Why? _____

EVENING

Physical Energy	Libido	Mind Mood
Blood Flow	I'm letting go of…	Challenges
Rest	Visions/Ideas/Seedlings	Artwork/Creativity/Ritual
Power	Wisdom	Inner Beauty

JOURNAL

NOTES

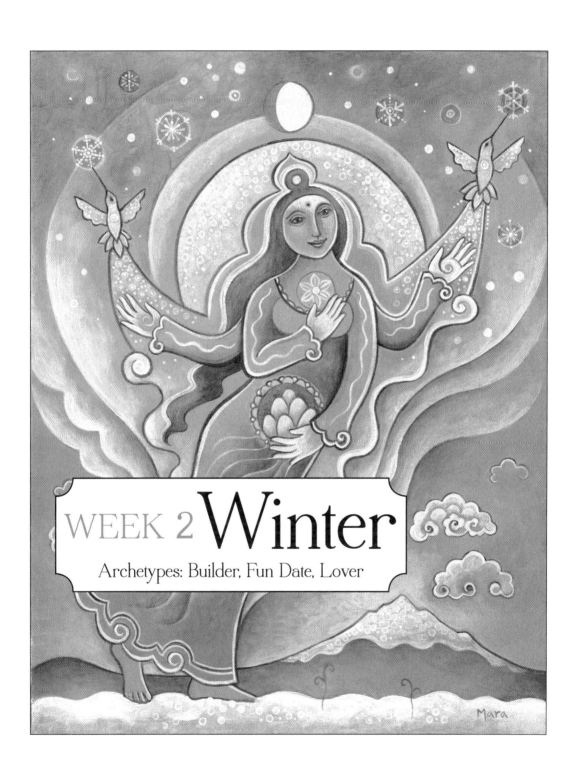

Daily Tracker — Week 2, Winter

Cycle Day:____ Date:_____ Focus: Become ❧ Connect ❧ Attract

MORNING

Woke up feeling: _____

Intention for the day: _____

Strength for the day: _____

Why? _____

EVENING

Physical Energy	Libido	Mind Mood
Heart-to-Heart Talks	Beauty Regimen	Challenges
Connections: People or Projects	Fun Outings	Obsessions
Power	Wisdom	Inner Beauty

JOURNAL

Daily Tracker — Week 2, Winter

Cycle Day:____ Date:_____ Focus: Become ❦ Connect ❦ Attract

MORNING

Woke up feeling: _____

Intention for the day: _____

Strength for the day: _____

Why? _____

EVENING

Physical Energy	Libido	Mind Mood
Heart-to-Heart Talks	Beauty Regimen	Challenges
Connections: People or Projects	Fun Outings	Obsessions
Power	Wisdom	Inner Beauty

JOURNAL

Daily Tracker — Week 2, Winter

Cycle Day:____ Date:_____ Focus: Become ✦ Connect ✦ Attract

MORNING

Woke up feeling: _____

Intention for the day: _____

Strength for the day: _____

Why? _____

EVENING

Physical Energy	Libido	Mind Mood
Heart-to-Heart Talks	Beauty Regimen	Challenges
Connections: People or Projects	Fun Outings	Obsessions
Power	Wisdom	Inner Beauty

JOURNAL

Daily Tracker — Week 2, Winter

Cycle Day:____ Date:_____ Focus: Become ❧ Connect ❧ Attract

MORNING

Woke up feeling: _____

Intention for the day: _____

Strength for the day: _____

Why? _____

EVENING

Physical Energy	Libido	Mind Mood
Heart-to-Heart Talks	Beauty Regimen	Challenges
Connections: People or Projects	Fun Outings	Obsessions
Power	Wisdom	Inner Beauty

JOURNAL

Daily Tracker — Week 2, Winter

Cycle Day:____ Date:_____ Focus: Become ❦ Connect ❦ Attract

MORNING

Woke up feeling: _____

Intention for the day: _____

Strength for the day: _____

Why? _____

EVENING

Physical Energy	Libido	Mind Mood
Heart-to-Heart Talks	Beauty Regimen	Challenges
Connections: People or Projects	Fun Outings	Obsessions
Power	Wisdom	Inner Beauty

JOURNAL

Daily Tracker — Week 2, Winter

Cycle Day:____ Date:_____ Focus: Become ❧ Connect ❧ Attract

MORNING

Woke up feeling: _____

Intention for the day: _____

Strength for the day: _____

Why? _____

EVENING

Physical Energy	Libido	Mind Mood
Heart-to-Heart Talks	Beauty Regimen	Challenges
Connections: People or Projects	Fun Outings	Obsessions
Power	Wisdom	Inner Beauty

JOURNAL

Daily Tracker — Week 2, Winter

Cycle Day:____ Date:_____ Focus: Become ⚜ Connect ⚜ Attract

MORNING

Woke up feeling: _____

Intention for the day: _____

Strength for the day: _____

Why? _____

EVENING

Physical Energy	Libido	Mind Mood
Heart-to-Heart Talks	Beauty Regimen	Challenges
Connections: People or Projects	Fun Outings	Obsessions
Power	Wisdom	Inner Beauty

JOURNAL

Daily Tracker — Week 2, Winter

Cycle Day:____ Date:_____ Focus: Become ☙ Connect ☙ Attract

MORNING

Woke up feeling: _____

Intention for the day: _____

Strength for the day: _____

Why? _____

EVENING

Physical Energy	Libido	Mind Mood
Heart-to-Heart Talks	Beauty Regimen	Challenges
Connections: People or Projects	Fun Outings	Obsessions
Power	Wisdom	Inner Beauty

JOURNAL

Daily Tracker — Week 2, Winter

Cycle Day:____ Date:_____ Focus: Become ❧ Connect ❧ Attract

MORNING

Woke up feeling: _____

Intention for the day: _____

Strength for the day: _____

Why? _____

EVENING

Physical Energy	Libido	Mind Mood
Heart-to-Heart Talks	Beauty Regimen	Challenges
Connections: People or Projects	Fun Outings	Obsessions
Power	Wisdom	Inner Beauty

JOURNAL

NOTES

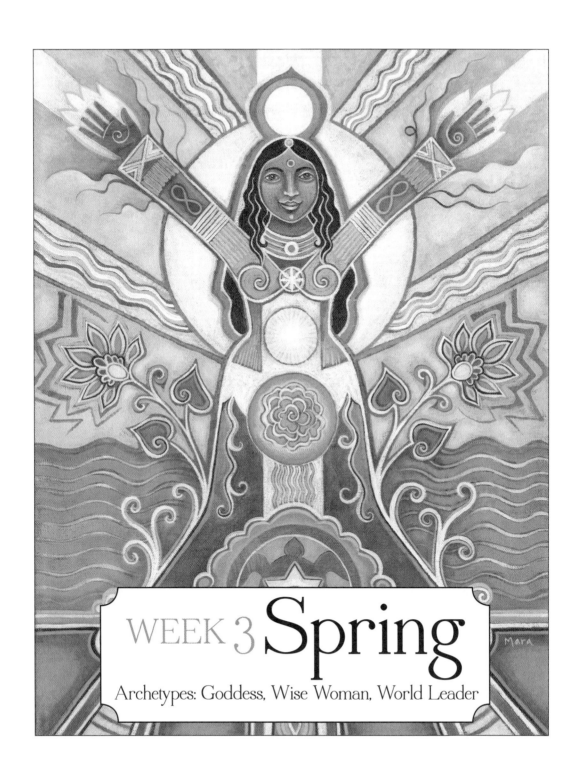

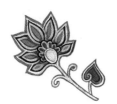

Daily Tracker — Week 3, Spring

Cycle Day: _____ Date: _____ Focus: Fully Express & Lead

MORNING

Woke up feeling: _____

Intention for the day: _____

Strength for the day: _____

Why? _____

EVENING

Physical Energy	Libido	Mind Mood
Full Expression	Vulnerability	Challenges
Authenticity	Mothering	Leadership
Power	Wisdom	Inner Beauty

JOURNAL

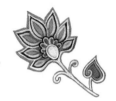

Daily Tracker — Week 3, Spring

Cycle Day: _____ Date: _____ Focus: Fully Express & Lead

MORNING

Woke up feeling: _____

Intention for the day: _____

Strength for the day: _____

Why? _____

EVENING

Physical Energy	Libido	Mind Mood
Full Expression	Vulnerability	Challenges
Authenticity	Mothering	Leadership
Power	Wisdom	Inner Beauty

JOURNAL

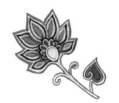

Daily Tracker — Week 3, Spring

Cycle Day: _____ Date: _____ Focus: Fully Express & Lead

MORNING

Woke up feeling: _____

Intention for the day: _____

Strength for the day: _____

Why? _____

EVENING

Physical Energy	Libido	Mind Mood
Full Expression	Vulnerability	Challenges
Authenticity	Mothering	Leadership
Power	Wisdom	Inner Beauty

JOURNAL

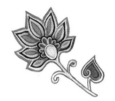

Daily Tracker — Week 3, Spring

Cycle Day: ____ Date: _____ Focus: Fully Express & Lead

MORNING

Woke up feeling: _____

Intention for the day: _____

Strength for the day: _____

Why? _____

EVENING

Physical Energy	Libido	Mind Mood
Full Expression	Vulnerability	Challenges
Authenticity	Mothering	Leadership
Power	Wisdom	Inner Beauty

JOURNAL

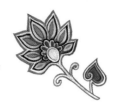

Daily Tracker — Week 3, Spring

Cycle Day: ____ Date: _____ Focus: Fully Express & Lead

MORNING

Woke up feeling: _____

Intention for the day: _____

Strength for the day: _____

Why? _____

EVENING

Physical Energy	Libido	Mind Mood
Full Expression	Vulnerability	Challenges
Authenticity	Mothering	Leadership
Power	Wisdom	Inner Beauty

JOURNAL

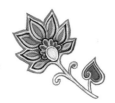

Daily Tracker — Week 3, Spring

Cycle Day: _____ Date: _____ Focus: Fully Express & Lead

MORNING

Woke up feeling: _____

Intention for the day: _____

Strength for the day: _____

Why? _____

EVENING

Physical Energy	Libido	Mind Mood
Full Expression	Vulnerability	Challenges
Authenticity	Mothering	Leadership
Power	Wisdom	Inner Beauty

JOURNAL

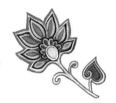

Daily Tracker — Week 3, Spring

Cycle Day: _____ Date: _____ Focus: Fully Express & Lead

MORNING

Woke up feeling: _____

Intention for the day: _____

Strength for the day: _____

Why? _____

EVENING

Physical Energy	Libido	Mind Mood
Full Expression	Vulnerability	Challenges
Authenticity	Mothering	Leadership
Power	Wisdom	Inner Beauty

JOURNAL

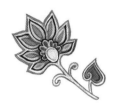

Daily Tracker — Week 3, Spring

Cycle Day: _____ Date: _____ Focus: Fully Express & Lead

MORNING

Woke up feeling: _____

Intention for the day: _____

Strength for the day: _____

Why? _____

EVENING

Physical Energy	Libido	Mind Mood
Full Expression	Vulnerability	Challenges
Authenticity	Mothering	Leadership
Power	Wisdom	Inner Beauty

JOURNAL

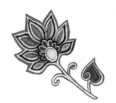

Daily Tracker — Week 3, Spring

Cycle Day: _____ Date: _____ Focus: Fully Express & Lead

MORNING

Woke up feeling: _____

Intention for the day: _____

Strength for the day: _____

Why? _____

EVENING

Physical Energy	Libido	Mind Mood
Full Expression	Vulnerability	Challenges
Authenticity	Mothering	Leadership
Power	Wisdom	Inner Beauty

JOURNAL

NOTES

WEEK 4 Summer

Archetypes: Athlete, Fire Walker, Monk

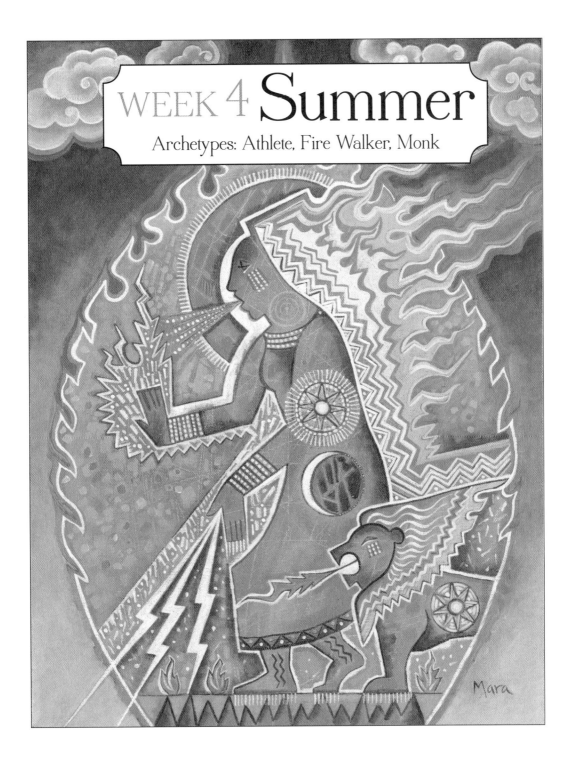

Daily Tracker — Week 4, Summer

Cycle Day:____ Date: _____ Focus: Exercise ❀ Observe ❀ Overcome

MORNING

Woke up feeling: _____

Intention for the day: _____

Strength for the day: _____

Why? _____

EVENING

Physical Energy	Libido	Mind Mood
Sports	Hot Spots	Challenges
Focus	I'm letting go of...	I'm keeping...
Power	Wisdom	Inner Beauty

JOURNAL

Daily Tracker — Week 4, Summer

Cycle Day:____ Date:_____ Focus: Exercise ❧ Observe ❧ Overcome

MORNING

Woke up feeling: _____

Intention for the day: _____

Strength for the day: _____

Why? _____

EVENING

Physical Energy	Libido	Mind Mood
Sports	Hot Spots	Challenges
Focus	I'm letting go of...	I'm keeping...
Power	Wisdom	Inner Beauty

JOURNAL

Daily Tracker — Week 4, Summer

Cycle Day:____ Date:_____ Focus: Exercise ❦ Observe ❦ Overcome

MORNING

Woke up feeling: _____

Intention for the day: _____

Strength for the day: _____

Why? _____

EVENING

Physical Energy	Libido	Mind Mood
Sports	Hot Spots	Challenges
Focus	I'm letting go of…	I'm keeping…
Power	Wisdom	Inner Beauty

JOURNAL

Daily Tracker — Week 4, Summer

Cycle Day:____ Date:_____ Focus: Exercise ✤ Observe ✤ Overcome

MORNING

Woke up feeling: _____

Intention for the day: _____

Strength for the day: _____

Why? _____

EVENING

Physical Energy	Libido	Mind Mood
Sports	Hot Spots	Challenges
Focus	I'm letting go of…	I'm keeping…
Power	Wisdom	Inner Beauty

JOURNAL

Daily Tracker — Week 4, Summer

Cycle Day:____ Date:_____ Focus: Exercise ❧ Observe ❧ Overcome

MORNING

Woke up feeling: _____

Intention for the day: _____

Strength for the day: _____

Why? _____

EVENING

Physical Energy	Libido	Mind Mood
Sports	Hot Spots	Challenges
Focus	I'm letting go of…	I'm keeping…
Power	Wisdom	Inner Beauty

JOURNAL

Daily Tracker — Week 4, Summer

Cycle Day:____ Date:_____ Focus: Exercise ❧ Observe ❧ Overcome

MORNING

Woke up feeling: _____

Intention for the day: _____

Strength for the day: _____

Why? _____

EVENING

Physical Energy	Libido	Mind Mood
Sports	Hot Spots	Challenges
Focus	I'm letting go of…	I'm keeping…
Power	Wisdom	Inner Beauty

JOURNAL

Daily Tracker — Week 4, Summer

Cycle Day:____ Date:_____ Focus: Exercise ❧ Observe ❧ Overcome

MORNING

Woke up feeling: _____

Intention for the day: _____

Strength for the day: _____

Why? _____

EVENING

Physical Energy	Libido	Mind Mood
Sports	Hot Spots	Challenges
Focus	I'm letting go of…	I'm keeping…
Power	Wisdom	Inner Beauty

JOURNAL

Daily Tracker — Week 4, Summer

Cycle Day:____ Date:_____ Focus: Exercise ⚜ Observe ⚜ Overcome

MORNING

Woke up feeling: _____

Intention for the day: _____

Strength for the day: _____

Why? _____

EVENING

Physical Energy	Libido	Mind Mood
Sports	Hot Spots	Challenges
Focus	I'm letting go of...	I'm keeping...
Power	Wisdom	Inner Beauty

JOURNAL

Daily Tracker — Week 4, Summer

Cycle Day:____ Date:_____ Focus: Exercise ❦ Observe ❦ Overcome

MORNING

Woke up feeling: _____

Intention for the day: _____

Strength for the day: _____

Why? _____

EVENING

Physical Energy	Libido	Mind Mood
Sports	Hot Spots	Challenges
Focus	I'm letting go of…	I'm keeping…
Power	Wisdom	Inner Beauty

JOURNAL

NOTES

Month

Cyclers: Begin at Period

Non-Cyclers: Begin at New Moon

Week 1, Fall / Period / New Moon / Rest/Vision / Internal	Week 2, Winter / Venus Week / Waxing Gibbous Moon / Become/Seduce / External	Week 3, Spring / Ovulation / Full Moon / Fully Express / External	Week 4, Summer / Fire Walk / Waning Crescent Moon / Observe/Transform / Internal	

Date

Day #	1	2	3	4	5	6	7	8	9	10	11	12	13	14	15	16	17	18	19	20	21	22	23	24	25	26	27	28	29	30	31
Low — Med O High +																															
Overall Health — O +																															
Energy — O +																															
Libido — O +																															
Mind Mood — O +																															
Sleep — O +																															
Communication — O +																															
Contraception																															
Sex																															
Exercise																															
Good nutrition																															
Beauty/Self-care 1-10																															
Feeling the Love 1-10																															
Indicators																															
Headache																															
Acne																															
Cramps 1-10 scale																															
Breast Tenderness																															
Irritability																															
Depression																															
"Hot Spots", Week 4																															

Keep Tracking!

Order Now at
4seasons4weeks.com:

*4 Seasons in 4 Weeks: Awakening the Power,
Wisdom, and Beauty of Every Woman's Nature*

4s4w Daily Two-month Tracker and Journal

The 4s4w Tracker Phone App

4s4w Refrigerator Magnets

The 4s4w ManGuide and other companion guides

4s4w Gift Items

And download a FREE full-size Monthly Tracker
and instructions! Choose between cycling
and non-cycling charts.

For bulk orders, please visit our contact page
at 4seasons4weeks.com.